Males With Eating Disorders

By Anthony Sepe

An Extensive Research Article
Male Eating Disorder Information & Recovery

 ISBN 978-0-9830670-2-3. Printed in the United States of America. For information, address Medical Nutrition Therapy Services and MaryLou Press, a division of AJ Sepe Enterprises, 16 St. John Ave G02 |Binghamton, N.Y. 13905|

Cover Design: Anthony J. Sepe

Dedication

Notes of Appreciation

This book is dedicated to all those with eating disorders, but in particular, males with eating disorders. This book is also dedicated to the memory of my Mom, Mary, and to my Dad, Louie, for their unconditional love and support of me. It is also dedicated to all my mentors – who by definition – are trusted friends who have believed in me: Betsy Rugala, RD, Denise Waters, RD, Dr. Joan Johnson, Dean, Sara-Jean Wagner, RD, Wendy Wolff, RD, Monika Woolsey, RD, Dr. Jennifer Bueche, RD, Dr. Nancy Collins, RD, Dr. Carlene J Ianuzzi, PhD, Dr. Jill Krilov, MD, Dr. Kevin Heintzelman, DO, Dr. Eric Hiester, M.S., DO, MD, Debbie & Brent Pickett, Margie & Ray Benza, Cindy & Mark Kostreba, Lisa S. Thomas, Michon M. Kerlin, Sarah M. McKeever, Sally O. Ondrejcak, Barry Goldstein and Dan Sheredy.

Males with Eating Disorders

Anthony J. Sepe, BS, DTR, AP4 Intern

DEFINITION of TERMS

Anorexia Nervosa (AN): -Characterized by a refusal to maintain a minimally normal body weight

Binge Eating Disorder (BED): -BED was officially introduced in 1992 at an International Eating Disorders Conference. The term was developed to describe individuals who binge eat, but do not use extreme compensatory behaviors such as fasting or purging to lose weight. In the past, these individuals were often referred to as compulsive overeater, emotional overeater, or known as food addicts. In the DSM-IV, Binge Eating Disorder is not an officially recognized eating disorder, but is included in the category titled, "Eating Disorder Not Otherwise Specified," as stated below. It is in a category for proposed diagnoses and includes diagnostic criteria to aid further study.

Bulimia Nervosa (BN): -Characterized by repeated episodes of binge eating followed by inappropriate compensatory behaviors such as self-induced vomiting; misuse of laxatives, diuretics, or other medications; fasting; or excessive exercise. A disturbance in perception of body shape and weight is an essential feature of both Anorexia Nervosa and Bulimia Nervosa.

Cognitive Behavioral Therapy ***(CBT):*** -CBT was originally developed in the late 1970's by Aaron Beck as a technique for treating depression. The term cognitive refers to mental perception and awareness. Cognitive distortions in the thinking of eating disorder patients that influence behavior are well recognized. A disturbed or distorted body image, paranoia about food itself being fattening, and binges being blamed on the fact that one cookie has already destroyed a perfect day of dieting, are common unrealistic assumptions and distortions.

DSM-III R: - Diagnostic and Statistical Manual of Mental Disorders, 3rd edition, revised

DSM-IV: - Diagnostic and Statistical Manual of Mental Disorders, 4th edition

Eating Disorders: -Characterized by sever disturbances in eating behavior

Eating Disorder Not Otherwise Specified (EDNOS): - This category is provided for coding disorders that do not meet criteria for a specific Eating Disorder.

MAIN PROBLEMS OR ISSUES

Weight issues have existed and concerned men for centuries. Because much of the focus concerning eating disorders has primarily involved women, men's difficulties with eating have escaped direct attention by society in the past. Recent stories of athletes' weight problems, juvenile self-image, and adult male body image help to focus the attention toward males' problems. The three principal disorders are the same as those that affect women and include anorexia nervosa, bulimia nervosa, and binge eating disorder.

Anorexia nervosa is a "voluntary, psychologically induced self-starvation"(l). It is also identified as refusal to maintain body weight at or above a minimally normal weight for age and height; intense fear of gaining weight or becoming fat, even though underweight; disturbance in the way in which one's body weight or shape is perceived; and amenorrhea in postmenarchal women for at least three consecutive menstrual cycles. In men, there is a decrease in sexual function and interest. Both restricting type and binge eating /purge type of anorexia exist (2, 3).

Bulimia Nervosa is described as recurrent episodes of binge eating. The term bulimia is derived from Latin and means "hunger of an ox." It is commonly known that the Romans engaged in binge eating and vomiting rituals, but it was first described in medical terms in 1903 in Obsessions et la Psychasthenie, where the author, Pierre Janet, describes Nadia, a woman who engaged in compulsive binges in secret."(4). A judgmental nature exists in this self-evaluation related to body shape and body weight. Two kinds of bulimia have been identified: in the purging type, self-induced vomiting or overuse of laxatives is typical; in the non-purging type, body weight is controlled by fasting or an overabundance of exercise, but the bulimic does not regularly engage in self-induced vomiting or the misuse of laxatives, diuretics, or enemas (2-7).

Binge eating disorder is identified as episodes of uncontrolled eating or bingeing (2) and is an "illness that resembles bulimia nervosa"(S). For example, a person might eat junk food for several hours, and consume an entire gallon of ice cream, or a whole bag of cookies, or the binge eater might do all these. It is reported by Carolyn Costin that the term binge eating disorder was developed to describe individuals who binge eat but do not use extreme compensatory behaviors such as fasting or purging to lose weight (4). In the past, these individuals were often referred to as compulsive overeaters, emotional overeaters, or food addicts. The bingeing characteristically separates the anorexics from bulimics. The bulimics are frequently labeled as failed anorexics--their weight issues are monitored by restricting intake and have been unsuccessful (4). It is important to note the position of the ADA regarding simple obesity. Simple obesity is included in the International Classification of Diseases (ICD) as a general medical condition, but does not appear in the DSM-IV, because it has not been established that it is consistently associated with a psychological or behavioral syndrome. However, when there is evidence to suggest that psychological factors are of importance in the etiology of a particular case of obesity, this can be indicated by noting the presence of Psychological Factors Affecting Medical Conditions (2,4). In other words, 307.50 is an Eating Disorder not Otherwise Specified. An "eating disorder not otherwise specified" (NOS) category is also provided for coding disorders that do not meet criteria for any specific eating disorder (7). Examples include:

1). For females, all of the criteria for Anorexia Nervosa are met except that the individual has regular menses.
2). All of the criteria for Anorexia Nervosa are met except that, despite significant weight loss, the individual's current weight is in the normal range;

3). All of the criteria for Bulimia Nervosa are met except that the binge eating and inappropriate compensatory mechanisms occur at a frequency of less than twice a week or for a duration of less than 3 months.

4). The regular use of inappropriate compensatory behavior by an individual of normal body weight after eating small amounts of food (ie, self-induced vomiting after the consumption of two cookies).

5). Repeatedly chewing and spitting out, but not swallowing, large amounts of food.

6). Binge-eating disorder: recurrent episodes of binge eating in the absence of the regular use of inappropriate compensatory behaviors characteristic of Bulimia Nervosa (2).

It is important to note, that the October 1998 issue of the Journal of the American Dietetic Association (JADA), The Obesity Epidemic: A Mandate for a Multidisciplinary Approach, discusses the implications of obesity and the importance of the integration of the physician, registered dietitian and support personnel in working with these individuals. (8). This paper will focus on the diagnosis of males with eating disorders, and treatments that have proven to be effective.

DIAGNOSIS OF EATING DISORDERS IN MALES

It is critical to include the viewpoint of the American Dietetic Association regarding nutrition intervention in the treatment of eating disorders, namely, anorexia nervosa, bulimia nervosa, and binge eating. The JADA contends that the etiology of the disorders are generally inclined to be present after restrictive dieting; however, only a small number of dieters' behaviors evolves into eating disorders. The individuals who do develop an eating disorder are susceptible to having the kinds of annihilating behaviors characteristic of an eating disorder (i.e., consuming unsafe diet nutritionals, following a trendy diet, desiring unhealthy weight ideals) (7).

Anorexia Nervosa

A male with anorexia often follows a routine diet that is restricted. For instance, the vegetables such as peas, carrots or lima beans are often counted. Exercise is very important to the individual with anorexia and much of the time normal exercise may become excessive in nature. The individual with anorexia generally develops a horror at the prospect of weight gain or the thought of being fat. Although weight loss is occurring, these preoccupations with thoughts about weight and about fat are not lessened. There appears to be a direct correlation between the decrease in weight and an increased concern over body image. The issue of body perception is paramount. It is known that most individuals with anorexia nervosa have a preoccupation with their appearance and weigh themselves frequently. In the diagnosis of anorexia, the type that is predominant must be determined. The clients with the restricting type of anorexia nervosa control their weight by dietary means and then continually exercise, as mentioned earlier. The clients who binge and then purge use a vast series of methods which include the self-induced vomiting, laxative abuse, and quite frequently the use of enemas to get rid of the food that has been ingested. The critical component for the diagnosis of anorexia nervosa is basically self-induced starvation. The anorexic has an intense fear of being fat, and this feeling is not in proportion to what it should be in reality.

In many instances, the anorexic individual will restrict intake of food and will also indulge in binge behavior, which leads to a classification of anorexia nervosa with bulimic complications or anorexia nervosa, bulimic subtype (ANB) (9).

These individuals are fairly easy to diagnose because of their body appearance. Physical signs of anorexia nervosa may occur in early to middle adolescence and include extremely thin or emaciated appearance (less than 85% of normal or ideal body weight), rapid loss of weight, loss of menstrual periods in women, growth of fine hair on the extremities, and frequent complaints of nausea, bloating, or constipation after eating normal amounts of food (10).

The food and exercise habits of the anorexic individual include cooking for others, yet, not for himself, being adamant about not consuming certain foods such as fat etc., refusing to eat, having an excessive concern about specific nutrients, indulging in excessive exercise, following a ritualistic behavior that includes cutting foods into small pieces, and being uncomfortable in social situation where food i's a part of the event (10).

The psychological significance and signs of anorexia nervosa include an unrealistic fear of weight gain and a feeling of being "fat"; an overall consuming attitude regarding food, weight, and exercise; perfectionism; minimal self-esteem; and being very lethargic due to malnutrition (10). In early medical sources, documentation of male eating disorders is virtually nonexistent. A literature search by Arnold Anderson, M.D. revealed only three case reports published in the 100 years between 1689 and 1790. There appeared to be speculation that these early case reports would satisfy the criteria that have since come to light regarding not only males with eating disorders, but eating disorders in general. It is felt that anorexia nervosa was indeed being addressed in early writing, but the situation was thought of as "a Nervous Consumption." (10).

Abraham and Llewelln-Jones report that anorexia nervosa occurs in males fifteen-times less frequently than in females. It begins in the same way, and its course is similar. Most males with anorexia nervosa are compulsive exercisers, spending long hours each day jogging, doing press-ups, and other exercises. They are as obsessed about food as women, but are less likely to show the same interest in cooking and cook-books. The authors further explained that men who develop anorexia nervosa may also binge-eat; an example is John who explained why he binge-ate: "Whenever I get worried about the fact that I have anorexia nervosa and that I binge-eat as well (and have to admit I vomit after the binge) my thoughts turn to Uncle Harry and His character, personality, and his periods of depression .... I do set my standards high, and it may explain my recent over conscientiousness and over consciousness -- an over consciousness of myself which has trapped me in a small world of self so that I have found it hard to work, to study, to relax, to sleep, to concentrate or even to communicate with others. I have become over conscious of everything I say and do" (11).

Bulimia Nervosa

Bulimia can be confusing and frequently intermingled with a subtype of anorexia. Males who binge and have been diagnosed with anorexia, should not be classified as bulimic, but rather, anorexic of the binge/purge type.

It is known that many individuals who are bulimic eat in secret. The food is usually extremely high in calories. Many individuals, eat a large amount of food in a short period of time, which is an amount definitely larger than most people would eat during a similar period of time and under similar circumstances. The binge is set in motion by many things; often hunger pangs from not eating for hours will set off the binge. There is a period of intense guilt arising from the bingeing. Because of the bingeing that has occurred, the client will often fast. The exercise routine may also start as a way to ease guilt and the uncomfortable feelings.

Relative to the diagnosis of bulimia nervosa, the bingeing complex must occur for a duration of at least three months. Many times the bulimic individual's body image is paramount to his self-esteem.

There are subtypes for bulimia. In the purging type, the individual is concerned with self-induced vomiting and laxative abuse; the body shape and the body weight are issues for this person. The nonpurging type individuals exercise and use periods of fasting, without purging.

In a Los Angeles Times article entitled "Silence and guilt" author Leslie Knowlton describes the enmeshed difficulties that males suffer as a result of their eating disorders. She explains that eating disorders have traditionally been linked to women, but "men also succumb to self-hatred and the battle to look good" (12). She further reports that "7 million women across the United States suffer from eating disorders, including anorexia nervosa and bulimia--life-threatening and often chronic illnesses for which exact causes are not known" and she continues "an estimated I million American men also struggle with the diseases" (12). Dennis Henning is 34 and suffers with bulimia. He has experienced a number of hospital admissions for his eating disorder. Prior to his fourth inpatient treatment program admission, he said his "mind was warped." Henning explains that food was like "land mines that catapulted him to binge and purge repeatedly, exercise compulsively, or starve for weeks"(12).

Binge Eating

Although binge eating may be associated with bulimia, there are episodes of bingeing not necessarily connected with purging behaviors, which are the main characteristics of bulimia. The client generally has no restraint and consumes food in great quantities until satiety is reached. The act of bingeing is done in secret, due to shame and embarrassment. For example, as reported by Ralph F. Wilps, Jr while he was in medical school "I would then carefully shop at convenience stores for 'just right' combinations of cheese, lunch meats, snack chips, and sweets such as chocolate bars. I would also make a stop at a neighborhood newsstand to buy escapist paperback novels (an essential part of the binge) and then settle down for a three-hour session of reading and slow eating until I could barely keep my eyes open. My binges took the place of Sunday dinner, averaging approximately 6000 kilocalories in size. Following the binge, my stomach aching with distention, I would carefully clean my teeth, wash all the dishes, and fall into a slumber." (9).

The requirements for this diagnosis are extreme distress during the binge as well as after the binge, and preoccupation regarding the after-effects of the bingeing on body weight and shape. The binges must occur for at least two days a week for six months. The November 15, 1995 issue of Patient Care, further clarifies the updated DSM-IV criteria for diagnosis of an eating disorder. It also more clearly defines "eating disorders not otherwise specified" than did DSM-111-R, and the new subtypes for anorexia and bulimia allow for more accurate descriptions. The DSM-IV asserts that "unlike the DSM-111-R, eating disorders exist on a continuum"(13).

David J. LaPorte reports that after observation of both the male and female binge eaters, it was the males who needed a vast amount of doughnuts or "rapid consumption" before the majority labeled it a binge, but women labeled much of their eating as a binge and experience dysphoria afterward"(13). He notes that gender differences are apparent because males were found to be feeling elated when the binge was completed. He asserts that this finding was more remarkable since a binge was typically defined for subjects in the study as intake of [greater or equal to] 4,000 kcals, (the equivalent of approximately 20 doughnuts), in the span of 1-2 hours (13). It appears that males are less inclined to be bothered by their bingeing episodes. Because male eating disorders tend to be seen on an infrequent basis, and because there appear to be stereotypic viewpoints concerning eating disorders in general, the male with an eating disorder will seldom receive a diagnosis.

It is known that eating disorders can often occur in males who are athletes. Those who, for example, need to hold their position in a certain wrestling class may be concerned with weight loss or gain in order to maintain a specific body weight. Swimmers are eager to be thin to improve their time, and their attention is focused on a slimmer body appearance. Both kinds of weight management carry with them an enormous amount of pressure. More frequently than not, a male will be concerned with his "physique" and maintaining "muscle tone" as opposed to the female counterpart who is concerned with what "size" she has attained. Cynthia Adams, says that there are varying groups of men who develop eating disorders, and in particular the "wrestlers, whom Adams calls the 'original bulimics' often vomit before weighing in and them gorge before the actual meet, setting up a pattern they cannot stop" (12). Dennis Henning, an individual with bulimia, reports that the suffering bulimic feels that "men are supposed to be men, and eating disorders are not something men are supposed to have ... if a woman asks for help, people say that's great, she's trying to bet better. If a man comes out with it, he's seen as pathetic" (12). Diagnosis is often changing in males because they have valid reasons for weight loss.to hold their position in a certain wrestling class may be concerned with weight loss or gain in order to maintain a specific body weight. Swimmers are eager to be thin to improve their time, and their attention is focused on a slimmer body appearance. Both kinds of weight management carry with them an enormous amount of pressure. More frequently than not, a male will be concerned with his "physique" and maintaining "muscle tone" as opposed to the female counterpart who is concerned with what "size" she has attained. Cynthia Adams, says that there are varying groups of men who develop eating disorders, and in particular the "wrestlers, whom Adams calls the 'original bulimics' often vomit before weighing in and them gorge before the actual meet, setting up a pattern they cannot stop" (12). Dennis Henning, an individual with bulimia, reports that the suffering bulimic feels that "men are supposed to be men, and eating disorders are not something men are supposed to have ... if a woman asks for help, people say that's great, she's trying to bet better. If a man comes out with it, he's seen as pathetic" (12). Diagnosis is often changing in males because they have valid reasons for weight loss.to hold their position in a certain wrestling class may be concerned with weight loss or gain in order to maintain a specific body weight. Swimmers are eager to be thin to improve their time, and their attention is focused on a slimmer body appearance. Both kinds of weight management carry with them an enormous amount of pressure. More frequently than not, a male will be concerned with his "physique" and maintaining "muscle tone" as opposed to the female counterpart who is concerned with what "size" she has attained. Cynthia Adams, says that there are varying groups of men who develop eating disorders, and in particular the "wrestlers, whom Adams calls the 'original bulimics' often vomit before weighing in and them gorge before the actual meet, setting up a pattern they cannot stop.

SYMPTOMS

Symptoms of depression are common underlying issues in eating disorders of both male and female. It is important **to** explore this and investigate how severe the symptoms have become. Self-esteem is often an issue and depression concerning the eating disorder itself can contribute to an already marginal self-esteem issue. Unsuccessful relationships and nutritional inadequacies contribute to depression. Many eating disordered individuals suffer from insomnia.

TREATMENT OF EATING DISORDERS IN MALES

Some characteristics of eating disorders are the same, regardless of gender, but there are other identifying features that are unique to males. The similarities and differences in treatment for males and for females with eating disorders are presented in the following chart from Anderson and Holman (15).

SlmUarlllit a d Dlffertn<to bt Treatment for Male• and Females Wllb Ealing Dlsordtts

Treatment	*Males*	*Females*
Nutritional Rehabilitation Sexuality	Testosterone supplement if needed Frequent focus on sexual role/ orientation	Estrogen supplement if needed Frequent focus on sexual abuse
Psychotherapy: Individual, group, family	Stigma from female eating disorder patients	Stigma from society for bulimia primarily
Treatment of medical comorbidity	Exercise for male muscle defmition, decreased abdominal fat, and increased bone density	Exercise for muscle to9ning, weigj:it distribution, and increased bone density
Treatment of psychiatric comorbidity	Consider same.gender therapist and group for some issues	Consider same-gender therapist and group for some issues
Relapse prevention	SSRis unproven for bulimia but logical SameforCBT	SSRI's proven for bulimia treatment SameforCBT

NOTES: SSRIF.Scleclive serotonin reupllke inhibitors; CBT= cognitive- behavioral therapy. (15)

Many professionals comprise the interdisciplinary care team including a registered dietitian (RD), physician, speech therapist, social worker, psychologist, psychiatrist, dentist, nurse and others as appropriate in overall treatment of the individual. As part of the team, the RD monitors the patient's progress as well as refers different medical problems to the appropriate health care individuals on the team.

A Better Way Health Consulting, Inc. explained in Recognizing Psychiatric Symptoms in a Nutrition Assessment that Psychiatric disorders alter cognitive perception of and response to stimuli (16). This alteration can create cognitive and emotional distress, for which the unknowing individual is likely to seek relief In many cases, the true reason for these cognitive distortions is abstract and vague. In an attempt to put some understanding to these feelings and distress, the client may visit a dietitian, thinking the distress is due to a dietary problem. It is important that the dietitian recognize basic sign and symptoms of a psychiatric problem, so that a referral for evaluation can be made. The diagnosis is always made by a psychiatrist or psychologist, never by the dietitian. However, the dietitian can be a crucial identification and intervention point for the individual who has not yet made the connection between their problem and a psychiatric or psychological explanation (16).

The American Psychiatric Association guidelines recommend nutritional rehabilitation as a first goal in the treatment of anorexia and bulimia. The guidelines do not address binge eating disorders. Since few therapists are formally educated in or choose to study nutrition, a registered dietitian or other individual specializing in nutrition education and treatment, is a useful and often necessary addition to the treatment team of individuals with eating disorders. Eating disordered individuals have a wealth of nutrition information and may often express an opinion that they do not need to work with a dietitian. Most often, their perception of their information has been distorted. For example, Carolyn Costin explains that knowing that "bananas contain more calories than other fruits becomes, 'bananas are fattening,' which becomes, 'if l eat a banana, I will get fat,' which means, 'I cannot eat bananas."(4). She further explains that a registered dietitian (RD) who has a degree from an approved program is the safest choice when looking for a nutrition expert, because the RD is the person who has been trained in the biochemistry of the body as well as extensively in the area of food and nutrition. Not all RD's are trained to work with an eating disordered client. It is known that most dietitians are educated and trained from a physical science standpoint. Dietitians are taught to investigate the protein, calories, vitamins/minerals and the variety of food intake. Most often this is seen as counseling a client, but in essence it is really nutrition education. Carolyn Costin points out that typically clients are educated about nutrition, metabolism, and even about the dangers their disordered eating behaviors could cause. They are also given suggestions and helped to see how changes can be made. For individuals with eating disorders there are two phases of the nutritional aspect of treatment: 1) the nutrition education phase of treatment, in which factual information is provided with no importance placed on emotional issues and 2) the experimental phase of treatment, consists of the RD having a special interest in long-term relationship-based counseling. The RD works in conjunction with other members of the health care team. All registered dietitians have the qualifications for the education phase, but to work effectively with an eating disordered client, RD's need to be trained in a psychotherapeutic counseling style (4).
The goals of treatment must include physical, spiritual, emotional, and cultural modification, rather than individually focusing on just one point in the recovery process.

An overall understanding will help the patient recognize how these different aspects correlate to food and weight related conduct. A comprehensive approach appears to be the method of treatment that males with eating disorders (or females with eating disorders) will benefit from the most. Although more research needs to be done on the specific psychological and personality features of males with eating disorders, the basic principles for treatment currently promoted are similar to those for treating females and include: cessation of starvation, cessation of binge eating, weight normalization, interrupting binge and purge cycles, correcting body image disturbance, reducing dichotomous (black or white) thinking, and treating any coexisting mood disorders or personality disorders. Such an approach requires focusing on the starting point rather that an ending point, dealing with the disorder and helping the family, as these members go through a tremendous amount of emotional pressure in most instances. Treatment may include antidepressant drugs, psychotherapy, and occasional inpatient hospitalization in some cases. Follow-up care is critical after inpatient treatment. Because susceptibility to relapse can occur, a compassionate approach is recommended. The philosophy behind this thought is to emphasize improvement as opposed to merely providing a quick cure. Part of the mechanism of treatment is that the recovered individual will emerge with a heightened awareness for undetected stress. Treatment is meant to help with recovery and will not present a real and immediate cure. Anderson says that "on the positive side, however, virtually every aspect of illness has the potential for substantial improvement or complete resolution" (9).

There are similarities to the treatment of eating disorders among males and females. In dealing with these treatment issues, professionals try to achieve an equilibrium effect between symptom decline and personal enrichment and growth, resulting in realistic views for the recovering persons with anorexia nervosa, bulimia nervosa or binge eating(9). The prognosis for males in treatment is comparable to that for females, at least in the short term. Long-term studies are not available. However, empathetic informed professionals are necessary, due to the fact that males with eating disorders feel misunderstood and out of place in society that still doesn't understand these disorders. Even worse, males with eating disorders are often made to feel uncomfortable and otherwise rejected by females similarly afflicted. Although it may tum out to be true, it is often mistakenly assumed that males with eating disorders, most particularly anorexia nervosa, are more severely disturbed and have a poorer prognosis than females with these eating disorders (4).

The ADA defines medical nutrition therapy (MNT) "as the use of specific nutrition services to treat an illness, injury, or condition. It involves the following phases:

(a) Assessment of the patient's nutritional status; and

(b) Treatment which includes diet therapy, counseling, and/or use of specialized nutrition supplements (7).

The process of medical nutritional therapy involves hard work on both the part of the nutritional professional and the person in recovery. They must work as a team to modify behavior. The process is difficult by nature and of extensive duration (7).

Many differing viewpoints come from a team approach with the best interest of the patient in mind as the end result. The treatment methods require frequent communication among the team members. For the treatment to produce desired results, the team members need to exist in union with one another and come to a consensus regarding what the patient's eating disorder is; they must also formulate a treatment plan that is mutually agreeable to all team members. The RD is instrumental in discussing the importance of treatment and recovery with both health professionals and family members involved in the recovery of the patient. When more than outpatient treatment is needed, further options need to be explored. Some options may include inpatient 24- hour hospitalization, partial inpatient treatment or a residential treatment center.

Anorexia Nervosa

In the past, males with eating disorders were expected to have less chance of successful treatment than females. However, current studies suggest that this expectation is not accurate. Today's professionals have found that the average male with an eating disorder remained in a thin-normal range of weight (92% Ideal Body Weight) and maintained considerable overall improvement in functioning during checkups six months to six years after treatment. Evidence suggests that successful treatment of males with eating disorders is possible, and case workers, family members and the patient, himself, should remain hopeful for a satisfactory solution to the eating problems (9).

The general medical consequences of starvation and the demoralizing and physically dangerous effect of purging behavior are not unique to either sex. On the other hand, the gradual, curvilinear return of plasma testosterone in the starved male, leading to increased thought of sexuality and the gradual return of sexual functioning, contrasts with the stepwise return of menses and reproductive hormone functioning in a woman who regains healthy weight.

Males, in general, need assistance in coping with a different kind of cultural pressure and stereotype than that faced by women with eating disorders. More often, men feel subtly or overtly under cultural pressure to achieve a classical male body shape, the inverted, triangular upper body. They become very self-critical when they perceive lack of adequate muscular definition of the presence of any "flab." They may be subjected to the demands of a "macho" culture in which they are expected not to show emotions, to be always strong, and to enjoy traditional male activities, such as working on cars and playing contact sports(9). Many males with eating disorders are uncomfortable with the stereotypical role but find it hard to evolve another more comfortable or acceptable role without feeling unmasculine or vulnerable to ridicule. Authors Dr. Arnold E. Andersen and John E. Homan, M. A feel that separate group therapy for males may be of benefit in regard to issues of stigma and sexuality. While most psychological symptoms of eating disorders can be treated in shared groups including males and females, males often feel stigmatized by eating-disordered females as well as by general society. Males with eating disorders feel misunderstood and out of place in a society that still sees this as a women's issue. In addition, females may be reluctant to speak about their personal sexual history or relationship difficulties with males when a male patient is present. Whether the gender of the therapist makes a difference has never been studied. Intuition suggests that during certain sensitive phases of treatment, a same-gender therapist may be of help. However, it seems to be beneficial to include members of both genders on treatment teams so that the individual with an eating disorder will feel comfortable with either a female or a male therapist. A core component of all inpatient treatment is early preparation for discharge and relapse prevention, a process that is relatively gender independent" (15).

Bulimia Nervosa

Treatment for eating disorders, and in particular bulimia nervosa, incorporates the use of antidepressant medication. An existing theory prevails that depression triggers anorexia and bulimia. Many research studies indicate and suggest the use of antidepressant medication in the treatment of bulimics. Substantial evidence exists and research outcomes have proven the demeanor of individuals with bulimia nervosa disorder can be helped by the use of tricyclic or selective serotonin reuptake inhibitor (SSRI) medications; however, while substantiated for treatment in females this is unsubstantiated for treatment in males 915). Researchers have found that this type of medication helps between 25 and 40% of patients to stop bingeing and purging 915). The most effective and most widespread method of treatment has long been cognitive-behavioral therapy, which helps even more people. Recent statistics indicate up to 65% of patients have stopped bingeing and purging" (17) with the use of this mode of therapy. Dr. Steward Agras wrote that a study of at least 75 bulimic patients had been successful one year after the end of their treatment because of a combined approach using cognitive-behavioral therapy and the use of antidepressant medication. He notes further that the psychotherapy was particularly effective in getting patients to stop purging, while the medication seemed to help decrease bingeing. The end result of all this indicated that the relationship should be client-centered and not therapist-centered. As a result, the therapist must be an active listener and must not dominate conferences by providing lectures. There needs to be a balance between the therapist and the patient for an effective therapeutic relationship (17).\

Binge Eating Disorder

Much controversy exists concerning the eating disorder diagnosis if the primary symptom is recurrent binges without vomiting caused by an individual that binges. This is now classified as an eating disorder not otherwise specified (NOS), but was classified in years prior as compulsive eating (9).

The RD has a major role in the treatment of binge eating, just as with the identification of anorexia nervosa or bulimia nervosa. The individual will many times go to the RD first for weight loss issues, and it is up to the RD to make appropriate referrals to other health care professionals. Frequently, the individual is noncompliant because of lack of understanding concerning the relationship between emotions and food. Dr. Gary Litovitz feels that "we are seeing a whole range of different types of eating that don't fit the classic categories." One of these patterns is the binge eating disorder (BED) in which, at least twice a week, people uncontrollably eat large quantities of food in a short time span but do not purge. They use binges to ease depression or anxiety, and then feel disgusted or guilty. According to the American Psychiatric Association, an estimated 30% of people who participate in weight control programs are believed to have BED (18). The concept of binge eating disorder is nothing new; however, this was commonly referred to as compulsive eating prior to the new classification in DSM-IV. There has been much controversy over the new classification because of the recurrent episodes of binge eating without purging. "The role of the Dietitian in the treatment of binge eating disorder is the same as for anorexia and bulimia nervosa"(7).

DISCUSSION

Experience working with patients with an eating disorder, reveals that food appears to be a symptom of a much larger problem - not the problem. While men may see their difficulty as a body-toning issue, women tend to see their difficulty as a weight issue. Nonetheless, most males continue with an unrecognized eating disorder related to food. The individual's recourse is to seek treatment primarily for psychological maladies, which need to be peeled away (as you would peel away the skin on an onion) before the eating disorder behavior can be addressed. The issues are hard to handle. As more research is conducted and more evidence is uncovered pertaining to the origin of problems for males with eating disorders, a regimen with be put into place for comprehensive treatment more readily available information regarding men afflicted with eating disorder.

CONCLUSION

Although the greatest concern about eating disorders seems to be addressed as women's issues, there is adequate evidence to suggest that this is also a problem for males. But males with eating disorders are still receiving less than an adequate share of attention. Despite the seriousness of the issue of eating disorders, it has only recently been recognized in males and should not be taken any less seriously than diagnosis in females. While most men remain eager to be fit and to be firm, they are not immune to anorexia nervosa, bulimia nervosa, or binge eating disorders. Gender differences exist secondary to the eating disorders themselves. However, these differences should not minimize the importance of recognizing the disordered eating patterns that may ultimately impact the individual, whether male or female, and lead to an actual eating disorder such as anorexia nervosa, bulimia nervosa, or binge eating disorders. The physical signs, food and exercise routines, and the psychological signs should all be evaluated for all these eating disorders.

REFERENCES

1 Platka-Bird, L. Class Discussions, Nutrition 140. SUNY Oneonta, Oneonta, NY. Sept. 14 and September 19, 1994. Medical Nutritional Therapy 341. April 28, 1997 and April 30, 1997.

2 Diagnostic and Statistical Manual of Mental Disorders. 4th ed. Washington, DC: American Psychiatric Association;1994;675,550

3 UIHC Eating Disorders http://www.uihc.uiowa.edu/pubinfo/estdis/paperla.html Assessed October 1998.

4 Costin, Carolyn The Eating Disorder SourceBook: A Comprehensive Guide to the Causes, Treatments, and Prevention of Eating Disorders.Los Angeles, CA; Lowell House:5,13,15,98,17-179,224-225,178

5 Position of the American Dietetic Association: The Obesity Epidemic: A Mandate for a Multidisciplinary Approach JAMDiet Assoc. 1998; Supplement S44

6 Andersen, AE .ed. Males with Eating Disorders, New York Brunner/Mazel Publishers; 199036 6 19-20, 137 40 393-394, 157

7 Disordered eating and Eating Disorders Anorexia Nervosa, Bulimia Nervosa, Binge Eating Disorders. Client pamphlet. The American Dietetic Association; 1997.

8 Abraham, S. and Llewellyn-Jones, D. Eating Disorders: The facts, 2nd ed. New York: Oxford University Press; 1987 53-54.

9 Knowlton, L. Silence and Guilt Los Angeles Times. May 23, 1995 v1 14,El,co3.

10 Diagnosing Eating Disorders What's New in the DSM-IV Patient Care Nov 15, 1995 v29,n18,93.

11 Laport, DJ Gender differences Imperceptions and [sic] consequences of an eating binge J Sex Roles: A Journal of Research. April 1997 V36, 479.

12 Andersen, AE and Holman, JF Males with eating disorders: Challenges for treatment and research: Psychopharmacology Bulletin 1997; 394-95

13 A Better Way Health Consulting, Inc. Eating Disorders Review September/October 1998.

14 Goldman, D. Eating disorder rates surprise the experts New York Times. October 04, 1995; cl 1.

15 Sagerman, C.A greater variety of eating disorders. Washington Post. May 03, 1994; v117sh16col 1.

TO NOTE:

The original work, *Males with Eating Disorders* by Anthony Sepe, has been used as a Literature Review for the Health Care Services Division Distance Education Sodexho Dietetic Internship AP4 Program, which was also posted on their website. On 12/05/2005, Google indicated that August 17, 2000, *Males with Eating Disorders* Information and Recovery, was listed on Eating Disorder Recovery Information at Poppink.com. According to Joanna Poppink, a licensed marriage and family therapist, private psychotherapist specializing in eating disorder recovery, Eating Disorder Recovery at Poppink.com is dedicated to offering support, inspiration, education opportunities for people with eating disorders and those who love them. The links of Joanna Poppink are for convenience only. Those pages from Google follow:

Web Images Grougs News Froogle **more»**

Google Anthony J. Sepe Search Advanced Search

Preferences

Web Results **1 -10** of about **15,200** for Anthony J. **Sepe. (0.18** seconds}

Male Eating Disorder Information and Recovery

... August 17, 2000. Males with Eating Disorders extensive article by **Anthony J. Sepe,** BS, DTR, AP4 Intern. Males with Eating Disorders ...

www.poppink.com/links/males.html - 19k - Cached - Similar pages

Honor Roll of Donors

... C. Newman Mr. Doug Nielsen and Mrs. Katherine A. Nielsen Dr. **Anthony** W. Norman and Dr ... Mrs. Marie E. Schultz and Mr. Garth A. Schultz Mr. Robert **J. Sepe** and Mrs ...

www.development.ucr.edu/indchancellorsassociates.htm - 20k - Cached - Similar pages

Honor Roll of Donors

... Rice Mrs. Lorna B. Rich and Mr. Elwood **M.** Rich * Mr. **Anthony** A. Richards ... Irene Ruibal

Mr. Christopher Sandoval Mr. Rob Schumacher Mr. Robert **J. Sepe** and Mrs ...

www.development.ucr.edu/indhighlanderclub.htm - 25k - Cached - Similar pages

Frank **Sepe** Nude Pies - Frank **Sepe** Naked Videos

... Daniel Stern Frank **Sepe Anthony** Stewart Nude, **Anthony** Stewart Naked ... Sam Elliott Nude,

Sam Elliott Naked, Clayton **J.** Barber Naked Frank **Sepe** Naked Roger .. ;

www.justcelebs.host.sk/Frank_Sepe.html - 24k - Cached - Similar pages

Renzo Cruz Nude Pies - Renzo Cruz Naked Videos

... Naked Renzo Cruz Naked Frank **Sepe** Nude, Frank **Sepe** Naked, David ... Rex Naked, Tony Bravo
Nude, Tony Bravo Naked, **Anthony** Kiedis Renzo Cruz Kevin **J.** O'Connor ...
www.justcelebs.host.sk/Renzo_Cruz.html - 24k - Cached - Similar pages
[More results from www.justcelebs.host.sk]

The Distinguished Flying Cross Society

... A. Selle, Albert L. Selleck Jr., Joseph **J.** Semanek, Donald M **Sepe,** Charles D ... Thomas A Shtogren, Robert P. Shultz, Michael L. Shuppert, **Anthony** J Siani, John R ... www.dfcsociety.org/honorroll. asp?offset=O&nav_letter=S - 84k - Cached - Similar pages

Official WOW List 1996-98 (wowzone.com) Wish Only Well

... Morgante, Margerita Rossi, Nancy & Donna Moore, Patrizia **Sepe,** Marsha Stanley ...
Annette
Ponto, Rita Santoro, Kim Lang, Joanie Murphy, **Anthony J.** Travis, Nancy ...
www.wowzone.com/wpeople.htm - 17k - Cached - Similar pages

Moraine Valley honors Blue Island man as 2003 Pacesetter

Eating Disorder Recovery at Poppink.com is dedicated to offering support, inspiration, education and treatment opportunities for people with eating disorders and those who love them. Please **see** ***our terms of use.***

Eating Disorder Recovery at

Poppink.com

These links are provided as a convenience only. This site and Joanna Poppink do not endorse, support or recommend any of the patties, services, products or other materials to which these links point.

Choose from Categories below

- Eating Disorder
  Treatment • Education Program
- Eating Disorder • Favorite Inspiration Site Information • Healthful Exercise and
- Males with Eating Body Awareness

	Disorders	Information
•	Nutrition	• Trauma Related Injury

Eating Disorder Recovery at Poppink.com is dedicated to offering support, inspiration, education and treatment opportunities for people with eating disorders and those who love them. Please see our terms of use.

Eating Disorder Recovery at Poppink.com

These links are provided as a convenience only. This site and Joanna Poppink do not endorse, support or recommend any of the patties, services, products or other materials to which these links point.

Choose from Categories below

- Eating Disorder Treatment • Education Program
- Eating Disorder • Favorite Inspiration Site Information • Healthful Exercise and
- Males with Eating Body Awareness Disorders Information
- Nutrition • Trauma Related Information
- Healthful Life & Treatment Opportunities
- Male Eating Disorders Information

Dr. Arnold E. Anderson, director, Eating Disorders Unit, University of Iowa College of Medicine, Iowa City, Iowa, e-mail: psychedinfo@uiowa.edu.

Submit a Site

Eating Disordersin Males
article by Leslie Knowlton in Psychiatric Times, September 1995, Vol. XII, Issue 9

Gender-Related Aspects of Eating Disorders: A Guide to Practice
by A1nold E. Andersen, MD
article in Journal of Gender Specific Medicine 1999;2[1]:47-54)

Male eating disorders canbe dealt with, once recognized
article by Kevin Beck in American News Service, August 17,2000

Males with Eating Disorders
Extensive article By Anthony J. Sepe, BS, DTR, AP4 Intern

Males with Eating Disorders
Edited by Arnold E. Anderson
This is the first book to chart this seldom documented territory. It Investigates the range of human needs that contribute to eating disorders, includes personal identity, body image, gender identity, gratification and impulsiveness, guilt, and even the physical demands of one's profession.

List of Articles on Eating Disorders in Gay Men

- Beren, S. E.; Hayden, H. A.; Wilfley, D. E. & Grilo, C. M. (1999, sep.). The influence of sexual orientation on body dissatisfaction in adult men and women. International Journal of Eating Disorders, v. 20 (2): 135-141.
- Brand, P. A et al. (1992). A Comparison of Lesbians, Gay Men, and Heterosexuals on Weight and Restrained Eating. International Journal of Eating Disorders, April, v. 11, n. 3: 253.
- Braun, Devra L.; Sunday, Suzanne R.; Huang, Amy & Halmi, Katherine A. (1999). Sexual Orientation and Eating Psychopathology: The Role of Masculinity and Femininity. International Journal of Eating Disorders, v. 25, n. 4.
- Cohen, Miles (1997). Eating Disorders in Gay Men - current issues. National Eating Disorder Information Centre

Bulletin, v. 12, n. 3: 1-4

- Duggan, S. J. & McCreary, D.R. (2004). Body image, eating disorders, and the drive for muscularity in gay and heterosexual men: the influence of media images. Journal of Homosexuality, v. 47, issue¾, 45-58.
- French, S. A.; Sto1y, M.; Remafedi, G.; Resnick, M. D. & Blum, R. W. (1996). Sexual orientation and prevalence of body dissatisfaction and eating disordered behaviors: a population-based study of adolescents. Inte1national Journal of Eating Disorders, mar.: 19 (2): 119-126.
- Gettleman, T. E., & Thomspon, J. K. (1993). Actual differences and stereotypical perceptions in body image and eating disturbance: a comparison of male and female heterosexual and homosexual samples. Sex Roles: A Journal of Sex Research, 29, 545-562.
- Heffernan, K. (1994). Sexual orientation as a factor in risk for binge eating and bulimia nervosa: a review. International Journal of Eating Disorders, v. 16, 335-347.
- Herzog, D. B.; Newman, K. L. & Warshaw, M. (1991, June). Body image dissatisfaction in homosexual and heterosexual males. J Nerv Ment Dis., 179 (6): 356-359.
- Herzog, D. B.; Norman, D. K.; Gordon, C. & Pepose, M. (1984, August). Sexual conflict and eating disorders in 27 males. Am J Psychiatry, 141 (8): 989-990.
- Meyer, Caroline; Blissett, Jackie & Oldfield, Claire.(2001). Sexual Orientation and Eating Psychopathology: the Role of Masculinity and Femininity. International Journal of Eating Disorders, v. 29, n. 3: 314-318.
- Russell, C. J. & Keel, P. K. (2002, April). Homosexuality as a specific risk factor for eating disorders in men. International Journal of Eating Disorders, 31 (3): 300-306.
- Schneider, J. A.; O'Leaiy, A. & Jenkins, S. R. (1995, Feb.). Gender, sexual orientation, and disorderd eating. Psychology and Health, v. 10 (2): 113-128.
- Siever, M. D. (1994). Sexual orientation and gender as factors in socioculturally acquired vulnerability to body dissatisfaction and eating disorders. J Consult Clin Psychol, April; 62 (2): 252-260.
- Silberstein, L. R.; Mishkind, M. E.; Streigel-Moore, R.H.; Timko, C. & Rodin, J. (1989). Men and their bodies: a comparison of homosexual and heterosexual men. Psychosomatic Medicine, 51: 337-346.
- Surgenor, Lois G. & Fear, Jennifer L. (1998). Eating

Disorder in a Transgendered Patient. A Case Report. International Journal of Eating Disorders, v.24, n. 4: 449-451.

- Williamson, I. (1999) Why are gay men a high risk group for eating disorders. European Eating Disorders Review, 7, 1-4
- Williamson, I. & Hartley, P. (1998) British research into the increased vulnerability of Young gay men to eating disturbance and body dissatisfaction. European Eating Disorders Review, 6, 160-170.
- Wood, Mitchell J. (2004) The Gay Male Gaze: Body Image Disturbance and Gender Oppression Among Gay Men. Journal of Gay & Lesbian Social Services, v.17, n. 2: 43-62.
- Yager, Joel; Kurtman, Felice; Ladnsverk, John & Wiesmeier, Edward (1988) Behaviors and attitudes related to eating disorders in homosexual male college students. The American Jom·nal of Psychiatry, v. 145, n. 4: 495-497.

Thank you to Adriana Nunan for providing the above list of articles. Adriana Nunan is a psychologist, specialized in Clinical and Social Psychology and currently writing a PhD Thesis on Internalized Prejudice among Gay Men.

e-mail is: adriananunan@adriananunan.com
Homepage: http://www.adriananunan.com

Return to poppink.com home page

Joanna Poppink, MFT, licensed marriage and family therapist, private psychotherapist specializing in eating disorder recovery, 10573 West Pico Bl. #20, Los Angeles, CA, (310) 474-4165

Joanna's professional affiliations

12J joann @poppink.com

Select a page from poppink.com here:
Home Go

LEGITIMATE NUTRITION
RESOURCE INFORMATION

American Journal of Clinical Nutrition

Nutrition Action

Environmental Nutrition

FDA Consumer

Harvard Medical School Health Letter

Healthy Weight Network

Journal of American Dietetic Association

Journal of Nutrition Education

Journal of Nutrition for the Elderly

Nutrition and The MD

Nutrition Today

Today's Diet and Nutrition

Today's Dietitian

**WEBSITES:
LEGITIMATE
NUTRITION
INFORMATION**

1. http://www.todaysdietitian.com
2. http://www. eatright.org
3. http://www.tufts.edu
4. http://www.medscape.com
5. http://www.vrg.org

About the Author

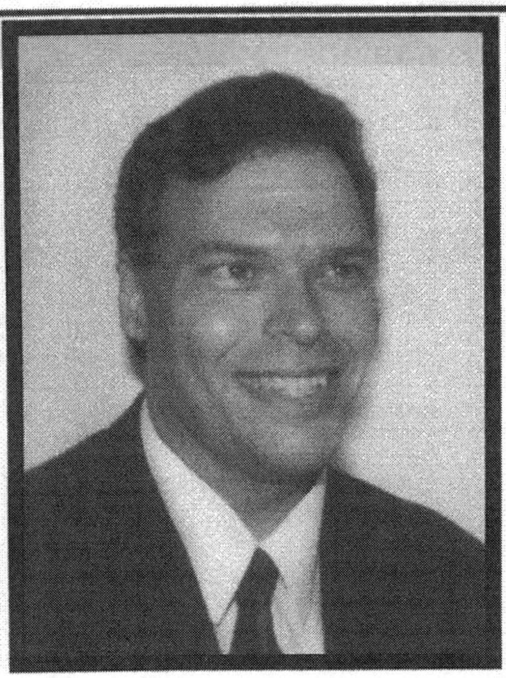

At the undergraduate level of education, Anthony was graduated in Science from Broome Community College; in FoodService Administration and Nutritional Care from the State University of New York at Morrisville, Morrisville, NY; in Dietetics from the State University of New York College at Oneonta, Oneonta, NY., and, at the graduate level of education, he was graduated from the Advanced PreProfessional Practice Program (AP4) Dietetic Internship Program through the Marriott Corporation - Healthcare Division of Sodexho Marriott, headquartered in Waltham, Massachusetts.

Made in the USA
Monee, IL
11 November 2026

67971454R00020